ACUPRESSURE FOR HEALTH

Effective Techniques For Pain Relief, Stress Reduction, And Wellness Enhancement Using Key Acupoints

DR. MELISSA STOTLER

Copyright © 2023 by Dr. Melissa Stotler

Disclaimer:

The data in this book, is solely meant to be informative and instructional.

This book is not intended to replace expert medical advice, diagnosis, or care. No medical, health, or other professional services are offered by the author, publisher, or any affiliated parties

Individual outcomes may differ in the practice of these therapies, which entail a variety of approaches and methodologies.

A one-on-one session with a trained or certified healthcare professional is still preferable. It is best to consult a trained healthcare provider before making any decisions regarding your health.

The author of this book is not affiliated with any specific website, product, or organization related to any of these therapies.

All reasonable measures have been taken by the author and publisher to guarantee the authenticity and dependability of the material contained in this book.

Contents

ABOUT THIS BOOK

Acupressure For Health offers a comprehensive guide to harnessing the power of acupressure to enhance well-being across multiple aspects of life. At its core, the book delves into the fundamental principles of acupressure, including an exploration of the body's energy channels and the strategic application of pressure through specific points. By understanding these basics, readers will gain valuable insights into how to effectively use acupressure tools and techniques, ensuring safe and effective practice while avoiding common mistakes.

The book's focus on stress relief highlights the key acupressure points designed to alleviate tension and promote relaxation. It presents practical techniques for integrating acupressure with breathing exercises, aiming to provide readers with a holistic approach to managing stress. Real-life success stories illustrate the effectiveness of these methods, offering inspiration and practical evidence of their benefits.

In the realm of sleep improvement, Acupressure For Health guides readers through targeted acupressure techniques that can enhance sleep quality. By examining how acupressure influences sleep patterns and incorporating it into bedtime routines, the book provides strategies to tackle common sleep disorders and achieve a more restful night's sleep.

Digestive health is another key area covered, with a focus on addressing common issues such as indigestion, bloating, nausea, and constipation. The book outlines acupressure points that promote digestive comfort and offers dietary tips to complement these techniques, supported by case studies showcasing improved digestive health through acupressure.

For pain management, readers will find detailed instructions on using acupressure to alleviate various types of pain, including headaches and back pain.

The book explores methods for effective pain relief and offers guidance on integrating acupressure with other pain management strategies, providing a well-rounded approach to chronic pain relief.

Mental clarity and focus are also addressed, with techniques designed to enhance concentration and memory through targeted acupressure points. Readers will learn how to incorporate these practices into their daily routines to manage mental fatigue and improve cognitive function.

The book's exploration of immune system support includes strategies for boosting immunity and preventing illnesses through acupressure.

By combining these techniques with a healthy lifestyle and adjusting practices according to seasonal changes, readers can strengthen their immune defenses and promote overall health.

Emotional balance is another crucial aspect covered, with acupressure techniques aimed at addressing emotional stress and anxiety.

The book offers strategies for emotional stability and integrates acupressure with mindfulness practices, providing a pathway to long-term emotional well-being.

Finally, Acupressure For Health helps readers create personalized acupressure routines by assessing their individual health needs, designing effective schedules, and tracking progress.

With resources for further learning and practice, this guide empowers readers to make acupressure an integral part of their health and wellness journey.

CHAPTER ONE

THE FUNDAMENTALS OF ACUPRESSURE

Acupressure is a technique rooted in traditional Chinese medicine that involves applying pressure to specific points on the body to promote healing and improve overall well-being.

This practice is based on the concept of energy flow, or "Qi" (pronounced "chee"), which is believed to circulate through pathways in the body known as meridians.

By targeting these points, acupressure aims to balance this energy flow and alleviate various physical and emotional issues.

Understanding The Body's Energy Channels

In acupressure, the body's energy channels, or meridians, are essential to understanding how the practice works.

These meridians are like pathways that transport Qi throughout the body, connecting different organs and systems.

There are twelve primary meridians, each corresponding to a specific organ or function, such as the liver, heart, and lungs.

Each meridian has a set of acupressure points, known as "acupoints," that can be stimulated to influence the corresponding organ or system.

For example, pressing on a point along the lung meridian may help with respiratory issues. Understanding these energy channels helps practitioners target the right points to address specific health concerns.

Key Acupressure Points And Their Locations

Acupressure points are located at specific spots along the meridians and can be accessed by palpating the skin. Some of the most commonly used acupressure points include:

LI4 (Hegu): Located on the back of the hand, in the webbing between the thumb and index finger. This point is often used for pain relief and boosting the immune system.

PC6 (Neiguan): Found on the inner forearm, about three fingerbreadths from the wrist crease. It's commonly used for nausea and digestive issues.

ST36 (Zusanli): Positioned about four fingerbreadths below the kneecap, on the outer side of the shinbone. This point is used to strengthen overall energy and improve digestion.

Knowing the exact location of these points allows for effective pressure application. Using a chart or guide can be helpful in identifying these acupoints accurately.

Tools And Techniques For Effective Pressure Application

Effective acupressure involves more than just pressing on points; it requires the right tools and techniques to maximize benefits. Some common tools used in acupressure include:

Fingers and Hands: These are the most basic and widely used tools. Use your fingers to apply gentle, steady pressure on acupoints.

The thumb, index, and middle fingers are most commonly used.

Acupressure Mats: These mats have a grid of small, spiked points that stimulate acupressure points when you lie or sit on them.

Acupressure Pens: These are handheld devices designed to apply pressure to acupoints with precision, often used for self-treatment.

When applying pressure, use a firm but gentle touch. Start with moderate pressure and adjust based on comfort and response.

Techniques include pressing, circling, or tapping the points. Ensure you are relaxed and in a comfortable position to enhance the effectiveness of the treatment.

Basic Acupressure Methods For Beginners

For beginners, starting with simple acupressure methods can help ease into the practice. Here are a few basic techniques:

Direct Pressure: Use your thumb or finger to apply gentle pressure on a specific point. Hold the pressure for 30 seconds to a minute, then release.

Circular Motion: Apply pressure to a point and gently move in a circular motion. This technique can help stimulate the point more effectively.

Tapping: Lightly tap the acupoint with your fingers. This can be a good method for stimulating points that are sensitive or tender.

Begin with one or two points and gradually incorporate more as you become more comfortable.

Practice regularly to understand how your body responds to different techniques.

Safety Tips And Common Mistakes To Avoid

When practicing acupressure, safety is crucial to avoid any adverse effects. Here are some important safety tips:

Avoid Excessive Pressure: Applying too much pressure can cause discomfort or injury. Start with light pressure and increase gradually if needed.

Consult a Professional: If you have any underlying health conditions or are pregnant, consult a healthcare provider before starting acupressure.

Stay Hydrated: Drink plenty of water before and after acupressure sessions to help flush out toxins and maintain hydration.

Common Mistakes To Avoid Include:

Ignoring Body Signals: Pay attention to how your body responds to the pressure. If a point feels painful or uncomfortable, stop and adjust your technique.

Inconsistent Practice: For best results, practice acupressure regularly rather than sporadically. Consistency is key to seeing improvements.

By following these guidelines and practicing regularly, you can safely incorporate acupressure into your routine and experience its benefits for enhancing your health and well-being.

CHAPTER TWO

ACUPRESSURE FOR STRESS RELIEF

Top Acupressure Points For Reducing Stress

Acupressure is a powerful technique that can effectively alleviate stress by targeting specific points on the body. One of the primary points for stress relief is LI4 (Hegu), located between the thumb and index finger.

Applying gentle pressure here can help release tension and promote relaxation. Another crucial point is PC8 (Laogong), situated in the center of the palm.

Pressing this point can ease emotional stress and calm the mind. GV20 (Baihui), found at the top of the head, is also beneficial for grounding and centering your energy, which helps reduce stress.

Techniques For Stress Relief And Relaxation

To maximize the benefits of acupressure for stress relief, it's essential to use proper techniques. Start by using your fingertips to apply gentle pressure to the identified acupressure points.

You can use a circular motion or steady pressure, depending on what feels most comfortable. It's helpful to apply the pressure slowly and steadily, gradually increasing it as you become more relaxed.

Combine this with deep breathing exercises—inhale deeply through your nose and exhale through your mouth.

This technique not only targets the stress points but also helps in calming the mind and body, enhancing the overall relaxation experience.

Combining Acupressure With Breathing Exercises

Integrating acupressure with breathing exercises can significantly amplify the stress-relieving effects. Begin by sitting in a comfortable position and focusing on your breathing.

Use your fingertips to locate and gently press the acupressure points identified earlier. As you apply pressure, take slow, deep breaths. Inhale deeply through your nose, hold for a few seconds, and then exhale slowly through your mouth.

This combination helps synchronize your body's physical and mental relaxation, providing a more profound sense of calm and reducing stress more effectively.

Recommended Duration And Frequency

For optimal results, practice acupressure for stress relief regularly. A good starting point is to spend about 5 to 10 minutes each session, focusing on the key acupressure points. Perform this routine at least once or twice a day. If you are feeling particularly stressed, you can repeat the process multiple times throughout the day. Consistency is key, as regular practice will help maintain lower stress levels and promote overall well-being.

Real-Life Success Stories And Testimonials

Many individuals have found relief from stress through acupressure. For example, Sarah, a busy professional, reported that using acupressure techniques on her LI4 and PC8 points helped her manage work-related stress more effectively. She found that incorporating breathing exercises enhanced her relaxation and overall stress management.

Similarly, John, a student facing exam pressure, used acupressure combined with deep breathing to calm his nerves before tests. His improved focus and reduced anxiety were significant, highlighting the practical benefits of acupressure in real-life situations.

These testimonials underscore the effectiveness of acupressure and breathing techniques in alleviating stress and enhancing quality of life.

CHAPTER THREE

ENHANCING SLEEP QUALITY WITH ACUPRESSURE

Acupressure Points To Improve Sleep

Acupressure can be a valuable tool for enhancing your sleep quality by targeting specific points on the body that influence relaxation and stress relief. One of the most effective points for improving sleep is the "Shen Men" point, located on the inner wrist, about three fingerbreadths from the base of the palm. Gently pressing or massaging this point can help calm the mind and prepare the body for rest.

Another important point is the "A Mian", situated just behind the earlobe, on the bone. This point is known for its ability to alleviate insomnia and promote a deeper, more restful sleep. To stimulate this point, use your fingertips to apply gentle pressure in a circular motion.

"Yin Tang", located between the eyebrows, is also beneficial for reducing anxiety and promoting relaxation before sleep. Applying gentle pressure to this area can help quiet the mind and ease you into a peaceful state.

Techniques To Prepare For A Restful Night

To prepare for a restful night using acupressure, start by creating a calming environment. Dim the lights and ensure your bedroom is a quiet, comfortable space. Sit or lie down in a relaxed position, and begin by focusing on deep, slow breathing to help reduce stress and prepare your body for the acupressure session.

Begin by applying gentle pressure to the Shen Men point, using your thumb or index finger. Apply steady pressure for about 1-2 minutes, then release and repeat as needed.

Next, move to the An Mian point and use your fingertips to apply light pressure in a circular motion for 1-2 minutes.

For the Yin Tang point, use your index and middle fingers to apply gentle, consistent pressure for 1-2 minutes.

As you work on each point, visualize calming and peaceful imagery to enhance the relaxation effect.

How Acupressure Affects Sleep Patterns

Acupressure influences sleep patterns by stimulating specific points in the body that are associated with relaxation and stress reduction. When you apply pressure to these points, it promotes the release of endorphins and other neurotransmitters that help regulate sleep cycles and improve overall sleep quality.

By activating the body's natural relaxation response, acupressure can help lower cortisol levels, the hormone associated with stress. This reduction in stress can make it easier for you to fall asleep and stay asleep throughout the night. Additionally, acupressure can help balance the body's energy flow, further promoting restful sleep.

Integrating Acupressure Into Your Bedtime Routine

Integrating acupressure into your bedtime routine can be a simple yet effective way to improve your sleep quality. Start by setting aside 10-15 minutes each night dedicated to your acupressure practice. Choose a comfortable, quiet space where you can relax without interruptions.

Begin your routine by performing deep breathing exercises to center yourself and promote relaxation.

Next, use gentle pressure on the Shen Men, An Mian, and Yin Tang points, as described earlier. You might also incorporate soothing music or calming scents, such as lavender, to enhance the relaxation experience.

Consider creating a consistent bedtime ritual that includes acupressure to signal to your body that it's time to wind down.

Over time, this routine can help condition your body to respond more effectively to acupressure and improve your overall sleep patterns.

Common Sleep Disorders And How Acupressure Can Help

Acupressure can be particularly beneficial for managing common sleep disorders such as insomnia, restless legs syndrome, and sleep apnea.

For insomnia, regularly applying pressure to the Shen Men and An Mian points can help calm the mind and prepare the body for sleep.

Restless legs syndrome, characterized by uncomfortable sensations in the legs that disrupt sleep, can also be alleviated with acupressure.

Stimulating the Liver 3 point, located on the top of the foot, can help relieve these symptoms by promoting relaxation and improving blood circulation.

For individuals with sleep apnea, acupressure may help by reducing stress and promoting relaxation, which can contribute to more consistent sleep patterns.

Although acupressure alone may not replace medical treatment for sleep apnea, it can be a valuable complementary therapy to help manage stress and improve overall sleep quality.

CHAPTER FOUR

BOOSTING DIGESTIVE HEALTH

Key Points For Digestive Issues And Comfort

Digestive health is crucial for overall well-being, and acupressure can play a significant role in maintaining it. This technique involves applying pressure to specific points on the body to stimulate energy flow and alleviate various health concerns.

To begin, it's essential to understand the common digestive issues people face, such as indigestion, bloating, nausea, and constipation. Acupressure can help address these problems by targeting particular points known to support digestive function.

Understanding the root causes of digestive discomfort is vital. Many issues stem from stress, poor diet, or irregular eating habits. Acupressure helps by promoting relaxation and enhancing the body's ability to process and absorb nutrients. By applying pressure to specific acupoints, you can help balance the digestive system, leading to improved comfort and overall health.

Techniques For Alleviating Indigestion And Bloating

Indigestion and bloating are common problems that can cause significant discomfort. To alleviate these symptoms, focus on acupressure points that help regulate digestive function.

Stomach 36 (ST36): Located about three finger-widths below the kneecap, just off the shinbone, ST36 is known for its ability to boost digestive health and reduce bloating. Applying firm pressure to this point can help enhance stomach function and ease discomfort.

Ren 12 (CV12): Found in the middle of the abdomen, Ren 12 is a key point for balancing the digestive system. Gently pressing this area can help alleviate indigestion and promote overall digestive comfort.

Spleen 6 (SP6): This point is located on the inner side of the lower leg, about four finger-widths above the ankle bone. ST36 can help reduce bloating and improve the digestive process by promoting the flow of energy throughout the body.

To use these points effectively, apply steady, moderate pressure with your fingertips for about 1-2 minutes each. This technique can be performed several times a day or as needed to manage symptoms.

Acupressure For Nausea And Constipation

Acupressure can also provide relief from nausea and constipation, common digestive complaints that can disrupt daily life.

Pericardium 6 (PC6): Located on the inner forearm, about three finger-widths from the wrist crease, PC6 is renowned for its effectiveness in reducing nausea. Gently pressing this point can help alleviate feelings of queasiness and improve overall comfort.

Large Intestine 4 (LI4): Found on the back of the hand, between the thumb and index finger, LI4 is another effective point for addressing digestive issues. It helps stimulate bowel movements and can provide relief from constipation when pressed firmly.

Stomach 25 (ST25): Situated on the abdomen, two finger-widths from the belly button, ST25 is beneficial for promoting healthy bowel movements and relieving constipation. Applying pressure to this point can help regulate digestive function and improve comfort.

For best results, apply pressure to these points for 1-2 minutes, using a steady, firm touch. This practice can be particularly useful when experiencing nausea or constipation and can be repeated as needed.

Dietary Tips To Complement Acupressure

While acupressure is a powerful tool for enhancing digestive health, combining it with dietary adjustments can maximize its benefits. Here are some tips to complement your acupressure routine:

Stay Hydrated: Drinking plenty of water helps keep the digestive system functioning smoothly and supports the effects of acupressure. Aim for at least eight glasses of water daily to maintain optimal hydration.

Eat a Balanced Diet: Incorporate a variety of fruits, vegetables, whole grains, and lean proteins into your diet. These foods provide essential nutrients and fiber that support digestive health.

Avoid Heavy, Greasy Foods: Foods that are high in fat and sugar can contribute to digestive discomfort. Opt for lighter, easily digestible meals to complement your acupressure practice.

Practice Regular Eating Habits: Eating at regular intervals helps regulate digestive function. Try to maintain consistent meal times and avoid overeating to keep your digestive system balanced.

By combining these dietary tips with acupressure techniques, you can enhance your digestive health and overall well-being.

Case Studies: Improved Digestive Health Through Acupressure

Several case studies illustrate the effectiveness of acupressure in improving digestive health:

Case Study 1: A patient with chronic bloating found significant relief after incorporating acupressure into their routine. Regularly applying pressure to ST36 and Ren 12 helped reduce bloating and improve overall comfort.

Case Study 2: Another individual experienced frequent nausea due to motion sickness. By using PC6 acupressure, they were able to manage their symptoms more effectively and enjoy a more comfortable travel experience.

Case Study 3: A person struggling with constipation saw improvements after consistently applying pressure to LI4 and ST25. The combination of acupressure and dietary changes resulted in more regular bowel movements and reduced discomfort.

These case studies highlight how acupressure can be a valuable tool for addressing various digestive issues, offering relief, and enhancing overall health.

CHAPTER FIVE

PAIN MANAGEMENT WITH ACUPRESSURE

Points To Address Common Pains

Headaches Acupressure offers a natural way to manage headaches by targeting specific points that can help alleviate pain. For tension headaches, applying pressure to the "Yintang" point, located between the eyebrows, can provide relief. Another effective point is the "Taiyang" point, found in the temples. Gently pressing and massaging these areas can help reduce the intensity of headaches and promote relaxation.

Back Pain Back pain can often be addressed through acupressure by targeting points along the bladder meridian, which runs down the spine. The "Shenshu" point, located on the lower back, is particularly beneficial. Applying steady pressure to this point can help alleviate lower back pain. Additionally, the "Yaoyangguan" point, located just above the sacrum, can be effective for both acute and chronic back pain. Regularly stimulating these points can support overall back health and reduce discomfort.

Methods For Effective Pain Relief

Identifying Key Points To achieve effective pain relief through acupressure, it's crucial to identify and target the correct acupoints related to your pain. Using a reference guide or app to locate these points can enhance accuracy. Apply firm but gentle pressure using your fingertips or a specialized acupressure tool. Hold the pressure for about 30 seconds to a minute, then release and repeat as needed.

Consistency is key, so practicing this regularly can maximize results.

Pressure Application Techniques Use the pads of your fingers rather than your fingertips to apply pressure. This helps distribute force more evenly and reduces the risk of causing discomfort. Employ a circular motion or a gentle kneading technique to stimulate the point effectively. Avoid applying excessive force, as this can lead to bruising or increased pain. If using an acupressure tool, ensure it is clean and suitable for your body's sensitivity.

When To Use Acupressure For Chronic Pain

Regular Sessions Acupressure can be a valuable tool for managing chronic pain when used regularly. Incorporating it into your daily routine can help manage ongoing discomfort and improve overall well-being. For chronic conditions like arthritis or fibromyalgia, targeting specific acupoints associated with these conditions can help alleviate symptoms over time. Aim for 15-20 minutes of acupressure per session, adjusting frequency based on your pain levels and response.

Monitoring and Adjusting Pay attention to how your body responds to acupressure over time. Chronic pain conditions can vary, so it's important to monitor changes and adjust your approach as needed. If you find that certain points are more effective or that new points need attention, adapt your technique accordingly.

Consulting with an acupressure practitioner or a healthcare provider can offer additional insights and ensure you're using the most effective methods for your specific needs.

Combining Acupressure With Other Pain Management Techniques

Integrating Therapies Acupressure can be combined with other pain management techniques to enhance overall effectiveness. For example, combining acupressure with stretching exercises can provide comprehensive relief for muscle tension and pain. Similarly, using acupressure alongside hot or cold therapy can target pain from multiple angles. Ensure that any combined therapies complement each other and do not interfere with the efficacy of your acupressure treatments.

Consulting Healthcare Providers Before integrating acupressure with other pain management techniques, consult with your healthcare provider to ensure compatibility and safety. This is especially important if you are using medication or undergoing physical therapy. Your provider can help you create a cohesive pain management plan that includes acupressure and other approaches, maximizing your chances of achieving effective and sustainable relief.

Understanding Pain Patterns And Response

Tracking Pain Patterns Understanding how pain patterns change over time can help you use acupressure more effectively. Keep a journal of your pain levels, noting any patterns related to activity, stress, or other factors.

This information can guide you in targeting the most relevant acupoints and adjusting your techniques. Tracking your responses to different acupressure points can also help identify which areas provide the most relief.

Adapting to Responses Acupressure responses can vary depending on the type and intensity of pain. Some points may provide immediate relief, while others might require consistent stimulation to show results.

Pay attention to how your body responds after each session and adjust your acupressure routine based on your observations. Adapting your approach according to your pain patterns can help you achieve more personalized and effective pain management.

CHAPTER SIX

ENHANCING MENTAL CLARITY AND FOCUS

Acupressure Points For Mental Sharpness

Acupressure can be a powerful tool to enhance mental clarity and sharpness. By applying pressure to specific points on the body, you can stimulate energy flow and improve cognitive functions. One key acupressure point for mental sharpness is Yintang, located between the eyebrows, also known as the "Third Eye" point. Gently pressing or massaging this point can help calm the mind and improve focus.

Another important point is GV20, located at the top of the head. This point is believed to invigorate the brain and increase mental clarity. To use it, place your fingers on the top of your head and apply gentle pressure in a circular motion. Both these points are accessible and easy to incorporate into your daily routine.

PC6, located on the inner forearm, a few inches above the wrist, is another acupressure point that can help with mental clarity. Applying pressure here can help balance your energy and improve your focus. Regular stimulation of these points can enhance your mental functions and overall cognitive performance.

Techniques To Boost Concentration And Memory

Boosting concentration and memory through acupressure involves specific techniques that target mental faculties. One effective technique is point tapping, where you gently tap the acupressure points with your fingertips. For example, tap GV20 on the top of your head and Yintang between your eyebrows for a minute or two each. This method helps to stimulate these areas, promoting better concentration.

Another useful technique is rotational massage. For instance, use your index finger to make small, circular motions on PC6 on your forearm.

This motion increases blood flow to the area and can enhance memory retention and focus. Combine this with deep breathing exercises to maximize the benefits.

Acupressure self-massage is also effective. Take a few minutes each day to apply gentle pressure to the key acupressure points while sitting quietly. Focus on your breath and relax your mind as you perform the massage. This practice can help improve mental clarity and concentration over time.

Integrating Acupressure With Study Or Work Routines

Integrating acupressure into your study or work routine can make a significant difference in your productivity and focus. Before starting a study session or workday, spend a few minutes performing acupressure on Yintang and GV20. This pre-task ritual can help clear your mind and prepare you for intense focus.

During breaks, apply pressure to PC6 to rejuvenate your mental energy. A short, two-minute session of acupressure can help you regain concentration and reduce mental fatigue. Consider using acupressure as part of your regular breaks, integrating it into your work or study schedule for enhanced efficiency.

For those who work long hours, try using acupressure techniques as a part of your ergonomic setup. Position yourself comfortably at your desk and periodically use acupressure to manage stress and maintain mental sharpness. This approach helps in sustaining focus and improving overall work performance.

Managing Mental Fatigue And Overwhelm

Managing mental fatigue and overwhelm through acupressure involves focusing on points that help relieve stress and restore energy. GV24.5, located just above the bridge of the nose, can be massaged to alleviate feelings of mental exhaustion. Gentle, circular motions on this point can help calm the nervous system and reduce stress.

Another beneficial point is ST36, found on the outer side of the lower leg, about four finger widths below the kneecap. This point is known to enhance overall energy levels and combat fatigue. Applying pressure here can help invigorate your body and mind, providing relief from mental overwhelm.

In addition, regularly stimulating LI4 on the hand, located between the thumb and index finger, can help reduce stress and boost your mental stamina. Incorporating this acupressure routine into your daily life can effectively manage mental fatigue and keep you feeling more balanced and focused.

Personal Experiences And Tips For Better Focus

Many people find acupressure to be a valuable tool for improving focus and mental clarity. For instance, some users report that incorporating GV20 into their daily routine has significantly enhanced their ability to concentrate and think clearly. They often recommend using this point as part of a morning ritual to start the day with a clear mind.

Others have successfully combined acupressure with mindfulness techniques.

For example, practicing acupressure on Yintang while engaging in deep breathing exercises can create a calming effect that improves focus. This combination can help users manage stress and maintain mental sharpness throughout their day.

For those struggling with mental fatigue, personal tips include setting aside specific times each day for acupressure sessions. Regularly incorporating these practices into your routine can help maintain consistent mental clarity and focus. Additionally, keeping a journal of your acupressure practices and their effects can provide valuable insights and help fine-tune your approach to boosting mental sharpness.

CHAPTER SEVEN

IMPROVING IMMUNE SYSTEM FUNCTION

Acupressure is a traditional technique that can significantly enhance immune system function by stimulating specific points in the body. By applying pressure to these points, you can help boost your body's natural defenses and promote overall health.

This section will guide you through the key acupressure points that are known to strengthen immunity, techniques to prevent common illnesses, and how to integrate acupressure with a healthy lifestyle.

We'll also discuss how to adjust your acupressure routine according to the seasons and share some success stories of individuals who have experienced improved immunity through acupressure.

Key Acupressure Points To Strengthen Immunity

Acupressure works by targeting specific points in the body that are believed to influence the immune system.

One of the primary points for enhancing immunity is LI4 (Hegu), located on the hand between the thumb and index finger. Stimulating LI4 is thought to boost overall immune function and reduce stress, which can negatively impact immunity.

Another important point is ST36 (Zusanli), located about four finger widths below the kneecap, on the outer edge of the shinbone. This point is known for its ability to strengthen the digestive system and enhance energy levels, which are crucial for a robust immune response.

GV14 (Dazhui), located just below the base of the neck, is another vital point for boosting immunity. Applying pressure here can help clear heat from the body and strengthen the overall immune system.

Lastly, PC6 (Neiguan), found on the inner forearm, about three finger widths up from the wrist, is effective in regulating the body's energy and reducing stress, which can further support immune health.

Techniques To Prevent Common Illnesses

Preventing common illnesses with acupressure involves regular stimulation of key points to enhance the body's resistance to pathogens. Start by incorporating daily routines of acupressure, focusing on points such as LI4 and ST36. To apply acupressure effectively, use your thumb or fingers to press on these points with moderate pressure for about 1-2 minutes each.

In addition to regular acupressure, you can use specific techniques to target illness prevention. For example, performing acupressure before seasonal changes can help prepare your body to fight off colds and flu.

Gentle, circular motions or tapping on these points can also stimulate energy flow and improve immune function.

To complement your acupressure practice, maintain good hygiene, stay hydrated, and ensure adequate sleep.

These habits, combined with acupressure, can enhance your immune system's ability to fend off common illnesses.

Combining Acupressure With A Healthy Lifestyle

Integrating acupressure with a healthy lifestyle creates a synergistic effect that can greatly benefit your overall well-being. Regular physical activity, balanced nutrition, and stress management are crucial components of a healthy lifestyle that supports immune function.

When combined with acupressure, these elements work together to enhance the body's natural defense mechanisms.

For instance, practicing acupressure after exercise can help relax muscles and reduce fatigue, while balanced nutrition can provide the necessary vitamins and minerals that support immune health.

Additionally, incorporating stress-reduction techniques, such as mindfulness or meditation, alongside acupressure, can significantly boost immune function.

Stress is known to weaken the immune system, so managing it effectively is essential for maintaining good health.

Seasonal Adjustments For Optimal Health

Your body's immune needs can vary with the seasons, and adjusting your acupressure routine accordingly can help maintain optimal health throughout the year.

During the colder months, focus on points that support warmth and energy, such as ST36 and GV14, to prevent seasonal illnesses and bolster immunity.

In spring and summer, when allergens and temperature fluctuations can affect health, targeting points like LI4 can help manage allergy symptoms and support overall vitality. In the fall, as colds and flu become more common, a combination of LI4 and PC6 can strengthen your immune response and enhance your ability to fend off illnesses.

By aligning your acupressure practices with the seasonal changes, you can support your body's natural rhythms and maintain better health throughout the year.

Success Stories Of Enhanced Immunity

Many individuals have reported significant improvements in their immune health through the consistent practice of acupressure.

For example, some have found that regular stimulation of ST36 helped them recover faster from seasonal illnesses and reduced the frequency of colds.

Others have shared that integrating acupressure into their wellness routine, along with a balanced diet and exercise, enhanced their overall energy levels and immune function.

These success stories highlight the potential benefits of acupressure in supporting a strong immune system and offer encouragement for those looking to improve their health through this ancient practice.

CHAPTER EIGHT

USING ACUPRESSURE FOR EMOTIONAL BALANCE

Acupressure can be a powerful tool for achieving emotional balance, helping to alleviate stress and anxiety and promote overall emotional well-being. By applying pressure to specific points on the body, you can stimulate the flow of energy and help restore harmony to your emotional state. Here's a guide to using acupressure to support your emotional health.

Points To Address Emotional Stress And Anxiety

When it comes to managing emotional stress and anxiety through acupressure, focusing on specific acupoints can be particularly effective. Some key points to consider include:

Yintang (Third Eye Point): Located between the eyebrows, this point is known for its calming effects. Gently pressing or massaging this point can help alleviate stress and clear the mind.

Shen Men (Heart Protector 7): Found on the wrist, in the crease where the hand meets the forearm, Shen Men is often used to calm the spirit and reduce anxiety. Applying gentle pressure here can help soothe the nervous system.

Neiguan (Pericardium 6): Located on the inner forearm, about three fingerbreadths above the wrist crease, this point helps to ease feelings of nausea and anxiety, promoting emotional calm.

Tai Chong (Liver 3): Situated on the top of the foot, between the first and second toes, this point helps to relieve emotional stress and regulate mood swings by harmonizing liver energy.

Techniques For Emotional Stability

Applying acupressure effectively requires a few simple techniques. Here are some practical steps to help stabilize your emotions:

Gentle Pressure: Use your fingertips to apply gentle, steady pressure to the chosen acupoints. Avoid applying excessive force; the pressure should be firm but comfortable.

Circular Motions: For a soothing effect, use circular motions when pressing on the acupoints. This technique can help enhance the flow of energy and relax the targeted area.

Breathing: Combine acupressure with deep breathing exercises. Inhale deeply as you apply pressure and exhale slowly, allowing your body to relax with each breath. This integration can amplify the calming effects.

Frequency: Regular practice is key. Aim to apply acupressure to these points several times a day, especially during moments of heightened stress or anxiety.

Combining Acupressure With Mindfulness Practices

To maximize the benefits of acupressure for emotional balance, combining it with mindfulness practices can be highly effective:

Mindful Breathing: As you apply acupressure, focus on your breath. Pay attention to the sensation of air entering and leaving your body. This helps to anchor your mind and enhance relaxation.

Meditation: Integrate acupressure into your meditation routine.

Begin by applying pressure to the acupoints and then transition into a meditative state. This combination can deepen your emotional release and enhance mental clarity.

Visualization: While performing acupressure, use visualization techniques to imagine the stress and negative emotions being released from your body. Picture these feelings dissipating with each breath and pressure applied.

Body Awareness: Tune into your body's responses during acupressure sessions. Being aware of how different points affect your emotions can help you tailor your practice to your specific needs.

Strategies For Long-Term Emotional Well-Being

For sustained emotional well-being, incorporate these strategies into your acupressure routine:

Consistency: Make acupressure a regular part of your self-care routine. Consistent practice helps maintain emotional balance and resilience over time.

Personalization: Pay attention to which acupoints work best for you and adjust your practice accordingly. Personalizing your routine can lead to more effective emotional support.

Integration with Lifestyle: Complement acupressure with a healthy lifestyle, including balanced nutrition, adequate sleep, and regular physical activity. A holistic approach can enhance the overall effectiveness of your emotional well-being strategies.

Professional Guidance: Consider consulting with a professional acupuncturist or acupressure therapist for personalized advice and advanced techniques. Professional guidance can provide deeper insights and support for your emotional health.

Testimonials: Emotional Healing Through Acupressure

Many individuals have found relief from emotional stress and anxiety through acupressure. Here are a few testimonials that highlight the effectiveness of this practice:

Sarah T.: "I started using acupressure to manage my anxiety, and I was amazed at how quickly it made a difference. Focusing on the Shen Men point helped me feel more grounded and calm. It's become a vital part of my daily routine."

James R.: "Combining acupressure with mindfulness techniques has been transformative for me. Applying pressure to the Tai Chong point while practicing deep breathing has significantly reduced my stress levels and improved my mood."

Emily K.: "Acupressure has been a game-changer for my emotional well-being. The Third Eye Point and Pericardium 6 have helped me manage my stress more effectively, and I feel more in control of my emotions."

These testimonials reflect the positive impact acupressure can have on emotional balance, offering hope and practical solutions for those seeking to improve their mental health through this ancient practice.

CHAPTER NINE

CREATING YOUR PERSONALIZED ACUPRESSURE ROUTINE

Creating a personalized acupressure routine can significantly enhance your well-being by addressing your unique health needs. Begin by understanding that acupressure, like acupuncture, involves applying pressure to specific points on the body to alleviate symptoms and promote healing. The key to an effective routine lies in customizing the practice to fit your individual health goals and conditions.

How To Assess Your Personal Health Needs

To tailor an acupressure routine effectively, start by evaluating your current health status and identifying your primary concerns. Are you dealing with chronic pain, stress, digestive issues, or sleep disturbances? Reflect on the symptoms you experience daily and consider how they impact your quality of life.

It may also be helpful to keep a journal of your symptoms and any related factors such as diet, stress levels, and sleep patterns.

Next, consult with a healthcare professional or acupuncturist who can provide insights into which acupressure points might be most beneficial for your specific needs.

They can help pinpoint the points related to your symptoms and advise on how frequently you should stimulate them.

This step ensures that your acupressure routine is grounded in a clear understanding of your health requirements.

Designing A Daily Or Weekly Acupressure Schedule

Once you've assessed your needs, it's time to establish a practical acupressure schedule. Decide whether a daily or weekly routine will best fit into your lifestyle.

For many people, a daily routine is ideal for maintaining consistent benefits, while a weekly routine might be sufficient for those with less severe symptoms or time constraints.

Start with short sessions, perhaps 5 to 10 minutes each, and gradually increase the duration as you become more comfortable with the practice. Allocate specific times of the day for your acupressure sessions, such as in the morning to energize yourself or in the evening to unwind. Consistency is crucial, so choose a schedule that you can realistically maintain.

Adjusting Techniques For Different Conditions

Acupressure techniques can vary depending on the condition you're addressing. For instance, if you're managing stress or anxiety, focus on relaxation points like those on the ear or wrist. For digestive issues, the target points to the abdomen and feet. Each condition may require different pressure techniques or point combinations.

Begin by applying gentle pressure to the designated points using your fingertips, and adjust the intensity based on your comfort level and the severity of your symptoms.

If you experience any discomfort, reduce the pressure or try a different point. It's important to listen to your body and adjust techniques as needed to ensure a positive experience.

Tracking Progress And Making Adjustments

Monitoring your progress is essential to ensure that your acupressure routine remains effective.

 Keep track of your symptoms and any changes you notice after each session. You might use a journal or a tracking app to record your observations and any adjustments you make to your routine.

Regularly review your notes to identify patterns or improvements. If you find that certain points or techniques are not producing the desired effects, consider consulting with a professional for guidance.

They can help you modify your routine or introduce new techniques to better address your evolving health needs.

Resources For Further Learning And Practice

To deepen your knowledge and enhance your acupressure practice, explore various resources. Books, online courses, and workshops can provide valuable insights and advanced techniques. Websites and forums dedicated to acupressure offer a wealth of information and allow you to connect with others who share your interests.

Consider joining local or online acupressure groups where you can exchange experiences and learn from others. Many resources also offer practical demonstrations and guided sessions that can help you refine your technique and stay motivated in your practice. By continually learning and practicing, you can optimize your acupressure routine and achieve better health outcomes.